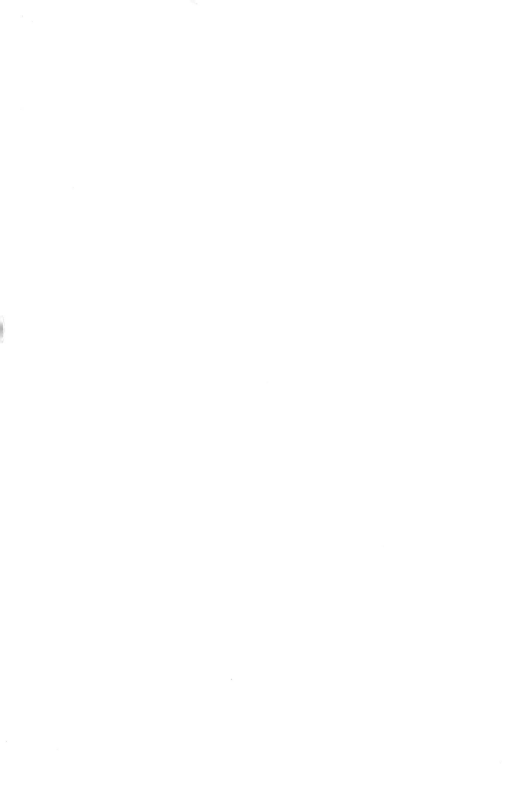

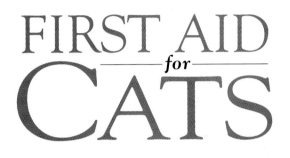

FIRST AID *for* CATS

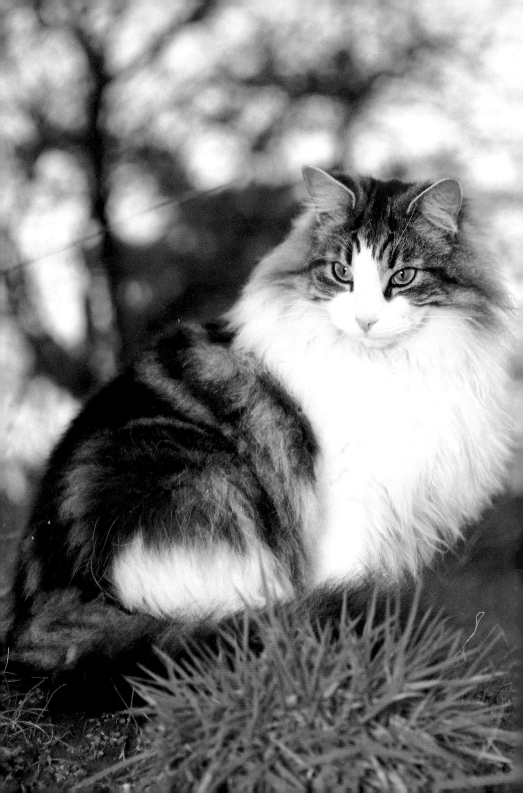

FIRST AID
—for—
CATS

The essential quick-reference guide

by

TIM HAWCROFT
BVSc *(Hons)*, MACVSc, MRCVS

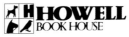

HOWELL BOOK HOUSE
New York

MAXWELL MACMILLAN CANADA
Toronto

MAXWELL MACMILLAN INTERNATIONAL
New York   Oxford   Singapore   Sydney

Howell Book House
Macmillan Publishing USA
1633 Broadway
New York, NY 10019

Maxwell Macmillan Canada,
Inc.1200 Eglinton Avenue East, Suite 200
Don Mills, Ontario M3C 3NI

Printed in Singapore by Tien Wah Press

Library of Congress Cataloguing-in-Publication Data:

Hawcroft, Tim 1946-
First Aid for Cats: the essential quick-reference guide/by Tim Hawcroft.
p. cm.
Includes index.
ISBN 0-87605-907-8
1. Cats - Wounded and injuries–Treatment–Handbooks, manuals, etc.
2. Cats–Diseases–Treatment–Handbooks, manuals, etc.
3. First aid for animals–Handbooks, manuals, etc. 1. Title
SF985.H38   1994   93-38167 CIP
636.808960252–dc20

Macmillan books are available at special discounts for bulk purchases for sales promotions, premiums, fund-raising, or educational use. For details contact:

Special Sales Director
Macmillan Publishing Company
866 Third Avenue
New York, NY 10022

Macmillan Publishing Company is part of the
Maxwell Communication Group of Companies.

10 9 8 7 6 5 4 3 2 1

CONTENTS

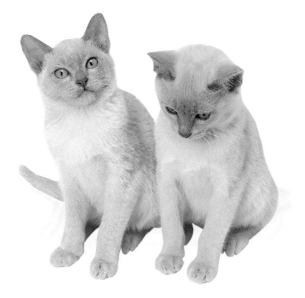

INTRODUCTION

This book of practical First Aid is designed for owners and cat lovers, in fact all caring persons, who want to know how to help a cat that is injured or sick, or who want to update and extend their knowledge of First Aid for cats. The know-how in this practical book, combined with experience, will give the reader confidence and skill to administer First Aid to a cat in most cases where there is a need for it.

You never know how, when or where you may be confronted with a cat needing treatment for some life-threatening, serious or simple type of injury or illness. You may already have come face to face with such a situation but been unable to help because of lack of First Aid know-how.

Road accidents, fights, hunting and the home are the most common situations where injuries and illness occur, ranging from fractures, abrasions, near drownings, cuts, bruises, diarrhea, bee stings and grass seed problems to collapse, hypothermia and severe bleeding. Usually, the injury or illness requires some form of First Aid. The increasing frequency of such injuries and illnesses in our community underlines a basic need for knowledge, skill and confidence in administering First Aid to cats as well as to other animals.

To save a life, arrest a worsening condition or just give some comfort and compassion to a cat in distress is a rewarding experience.

THE CONCEPT OF FIRST AID

When a cat is hurt or sick, many people do not know how to help. It may be because they do not know how to approach and handle a cat or they do not know how to administer First Aid.

First Aid is not a new concept. Cat owners and others have been practising it for generations. First Aid information has been passed around mainly by word of mouth, but in recent times the media, authors, veterinarians and cat clubs have been disseminating it. The most practical understanding of the term is in its literal interpretation: it is the *First* Aid, help or treatment that is given to an injured or sick cat.

Minor, uncomplicated problems such as a bee sting, grass seed penetration or simple cuts and abrasions may only need a single treatment or, at the most, repetitions of it. The treatment starts and finishes on-site or at home.

Serious and life-threatening injuries and sickness, such as fractures, arterial bleeding, self-mutilation and poisoning, need not only immediate First Aid but require further treatment by a veterinarian.

When an injury or sickness occurs at home or, for example, on a roadway in the case of a car accident, there is usually no veterinarian present. Whatever First Aid is given depends on the knowledge, skill, initiative and confidence of the owner or onlooker and the nature of the cat's injury or sickness. First Aid may range from something very simple, such as comforting the cat, to assessing its condition, perhaps moving it to safety, and then giving it the treatment thought necessary at the time.

Remember that *First* Aid is the first treatment and whatever treatment you can give is better than none at all.

HOW TO USE THIS BOOK

Familiarise yourself with the book's design, the location of various sections and their content. In doing so, you will be able to refer to the book for information in a calm, confident and speedy manner, especially in emergency situations. For ease of reference, we have set out the techniques, injuries and illnesses in alphabetical order. A detailed index in the back of the book will quickly guide you to the information you need.

Of course, the information you require will depend on the situation and your knowledge. You will have to use your own judgement to determine your course of action.

If you are in a situation where a cat requires First Aid and you are unsure of the action you should take, we suggest you refer to the following sections in this order:
1. First Aid Priorities (see page 13)
2. The Injured Cat(see page 14)
3. When To Call Your Veterinarian (see page 21)
4. First Aid for Injuries and Illness (see page 48)

These sections offer practical guidance and back-up information so that you can determine what procedure to adopt to treat a particular injury or illness.

Although this book will serve you well in an emergency situation, it is best to be prepared. The purpose of the First Aid Kit section is to prompt you to set up a First Aid kit of your own. Likewise the section on Accident Prevention is there to remind you of the old adage: prevention is better than cure.

To achieve competence in any activity involving skill you must practise. The sections dealing with the Injured Cat and Techniques You Should Know contain procedures you should learn. The more you practise and the closer that practice is to reality, the more proficient and confident you will be when facing a real life situation.

IMPORTANT
Always keep your veterinarian's telephone number handy.

ACCIDENT PREVENTION

CAR SAFETY

• Never drive or travel in a car with a cat sitting on your lap or on the seat. The cat could very easily become frightened, jump onto the driver and cause an accident.

• Use a carry cage or basket to contain the cat. Do not use a cardboard box as the cat may escape or, if the cat becomes terrified, may claw a way out.

• In some countries it is an offence to drive with your cat if the cat is not confined in a carry cage or basket.

• If you have to leave your cat in the car on a hot summer's day, make sure that the car is parked in a cool spot and that the windows are down slightly to allow some airflow.

• Before leaving on a long journey, restrict the cat's food and water intake for two to three hours. In hot weather, the cat will need to have a drink now and then throughout the day.

ELECTRICAL APPLIANCES

• Take care with electrical cords. Kittens and young cats like playing with moving objects. For instance, an electrical cord attached to an iron or a lawn mower, dangling or wriggling along the ground, is attractive enough for the young kitten or cat to bite in play. If the cat's teeth penetrate the plastic covering, electric shock will result.

• If you use a blow-drier after shampooing your cat, make sure that the appliance does not accidentally fall into the water. Do not rest the drier on the side of the tub whilst the cat is standing in the water.

POISONS

• Cats are natural foragers. Do not leave contaminated food, garden pest pellets and sprays, weed killers and the like exposed and accessible to a hungry or thirsty cat, whether your own or another owner's.

• Never let your cat roam. The free-roaming cat is subject to road accidents, fight wounds and serious illnesses.

ROAMING

• If you or your neighbour own a pool, take your cat into the water and show it where to get out. Make sure that your cat has sufficient practice in getting out of the pool and knows what to do in the water when no one is around to help.

SWIMMING POOLS

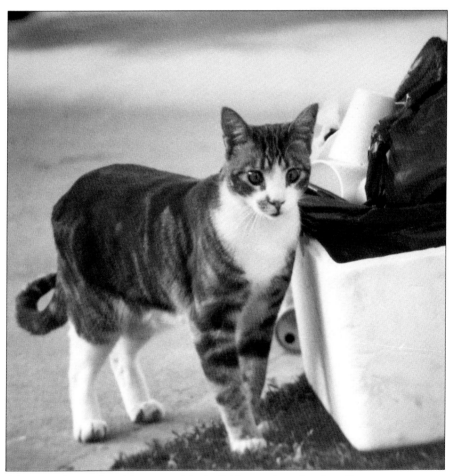

A free-roaming cat is subject to accidents, fight wounds and serious illnesses.

11

FIRST AID KIT

• Store the First Aid kit in a suitable container, readily accessible, portable and marked for easy identification.

• Clean any soiled instruments after use and if necessary restock the kit.

• Every six months check the kit to see that everything is in good working order; for example, test the torch (flashlight) batteries.

• The kit should include the following items:

- Antibiotic powder

- Antiseptic wash

- Eye dropper

- Gauze swabs

- Hydrogen peroxide 3%

- Mercurochrome (antiseptic solution)

- Paraffin oil

- Roll of cottonwool (absorbent cotton)

- Roll of adhesive bandage (2.5cm (1in) or 7.5cm (3in) wide)

- Roll of gauze bandage (2.5cm (1in) wide)

- Scissors (sharp, pointed, 10cm (4in) long)

- Syringe (plastic, 20ml)

- Thermometer (same as for human use)

- Tincture of iodine (anti-bacterial, anti-fungal solution)

- Torch (flashlight)

- Tweezers (forceps)

- Vetwrap bandage

FIRST AID PRIORITIES

- Keep calm and work methodically.
- Assess whether injury or illness is life-threatening.
- In any severe or critical injury or illness, treat for shock by keeping the cat quiet and warm (see page 86).

1. Life-threatening injuries or illness

First treat life-threatening conditions, with such signs as:
- Severe bleeding (blood pulsating or flowing freely from wound) (see page 58).
- No sign of breathing (see page 44).
- No heartbeat (pulse) (see page 31 and 44).

2. Non-life-threatening injuries or illness accompanied by severe pain

Next treat injuries or illness, such as a fracture or extensive burn, which are causing severe pain but are not life-threatening.
Approach with caution.
Your treatment concerns both preventing the injury from worsening and preparing the cat for transportation to the veterinarian.

3. Minor injuries or illness

Injuries or illness such as a slight abrasion or cut come last in the order of priorities for treatment.
Treat the cat at home if you know how.
Take the cat to the veterinarian if the injury worsens, for example, if signs of inflammation develop and/or the cat develops a temperature.

THE INJURED CAT

Approaching, Calming, Handling, Assessing, Lifting and Carrying, Holding

APPROACHING

• Approach an injured cat with caution as a cat that is frightened or in pain may attempt to bite or scratch.

• Before touching the cat, check for the following signs:

- The cat is conscious or unconscious (see page 15).
- The cat is bleeding (see page 58) or there is blood on the ground.
- There are obvious wounds (see page 87) or broken bones (see page 70).
- The cat's breathing is normal or laboured, rapid, shallow or absent (see page 44).
- The cat appears to be in a state of shock (see page 86).
- The cat is aggressive, most often indicated by hissing with mouth open, baring of teeth, drawn-back ears, dilated pupils, or erect hair on the cat's back.

CALMING

• Be cautious when calming an injured cat as, depending on the nature of the injury and the cat's disposition, you may be bitten or scratched if you touch the injured area.

• Talk to the cat quietly and soothingly. If there are no signs of aggression, stroke the cat. This is a soft, calm action unlike patting which may disturb the cat and provoke an aggressive reaction.

• If immobile, see that the cat is in a comfortable position. If moving around excitedly, confine the cat in a small space in the company of a reassuring person.

• If the cat appears to be cold, for example, shivering and shaking, put a blanket or rug over or around the cat's body.
• If the cat appears to be excessively hot, for example, panting vigorously and rapidly, use a fan or an icepack to cool the cat down.

If the cat is unconscious and breathing

HANDLING

• Roll the cat over onto the right side with the head tilted backwards and in a position lower than the rest of the body. Advantages of this position are:

- It opens up the airway.
- It prevents the tongue obstructing the airway.
- Vomit, fluid and foreign material will drain out of the mouth.
- It makes it easier to observe and check the cat's breathing and heartbeat.

• Cover the cat with a blanket or towel to help maintain normal body temperature. The cover should not restrict breathing or make it difficult to check breathing or circulation (colour of gums and tongue, heartbeat), or other injuries.

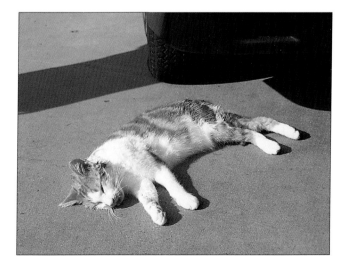

Place an unconscious cat onto the right side.

If the cat is unconscious, not breathing, and perhaps has a blue tongue

• Apply resuscitation immediately (see page 44) and check for severe bleeding before making any further assessment.

If the cat is conscious and aggressive

• Do not touch the cat.
• Take a blanket or towel in your hands, talk to the cat reassuringly, and quickly but gently place the cover completely over and around the cat.
• Touch the cover around the head of the cat to assess the reaction.
• If the cat does not appear to be aggressive, take hold of the still covered cat with both hands behind the shoulders and lift the cat into a suitable cat basket or cage from which there is no escape.
• Take the cat to your veterinarian.
• If no suitable basket or cage is available, ensure the cat is securely wrapped before transporting to your veterinarian (see page 20 for diagram).

If the cat is conscious and not aggressive

• Rub the back of your hand behind the cat's ears and then turn your hand to take a good handful of the scruff of its neck. This grip gives you good control of the cat, particularly the head.
• Then assess the cat's condition.

ASSESSING THE CAT'S CONDITION

Look at the colour of the gums

• If the gums are pale or white and there is no sign of severe external bleeding, the cat is probably suffering from shock (see page 86) or internal blood loss. Take the cat to the veterinarian immediately.
• If the gums are pink, it is a good sign that there is no major blood loss externally or internally.

Carefully run your free hand over the cat's body

• Look and feel for a wound, swelling or painful area.
• Check the movement of the limbs and note if there
is pain, swelling, a grating sensation or a floppy limb
irregular in appearance. Note if the cat itself cannot move
one or more of its limbs. These signs indicate that the
limb, pelvis or spine may be broken (fractured) (see page
70) or the joint dislocated.

Prop the cat up on four legs and encourage the cat to walk

• If the cat flops down, walks on three legs and carries
the fourth, limps, staggers, refuses to move, cries
frequently as if in pain or breathes in a laboured panting
fashion, wrap the cat in a blanket for warmth and to
counteract shock and visit the veterinarian immediately.

If the cat is able to stand but reluctant to walk

• *If a forelimb is injured,* lift the cat by holding the scruff
of the neck in one hand and support the body by
cupping the other hand around the hindquarters
(see page 18).
• *If a hind limb or pelvis is injured,* lift the cat by holding
the scruff of the neck in one hand and support the body
by placing the other hand under the chest (see page 19).

If the cat is unable to stand

• Improvise a stretcher by placing a towel, coat or folded
rug or blanket on the ground next to the injured cat.
• Take the cat by the scruff of the neck in a firm grip and
pull it on to the improvised stretcher.
• One person takes hold of the corners of the stretcher at
one end whilst another person holds the corners at the
other end (see page 19).
• Lift and carry the cat to safety nearby, then home or to
a car for transportation to a veterinary hospital.

LIFTING AND CARRYING

When assessing injuries look for signs like a cat standing on three legs and carrying the fourth which may be broken.

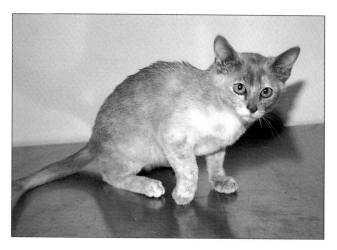

To carry a cat with a fractured forelimb, hold the scruff of the neck and support the body under the hindquarters.

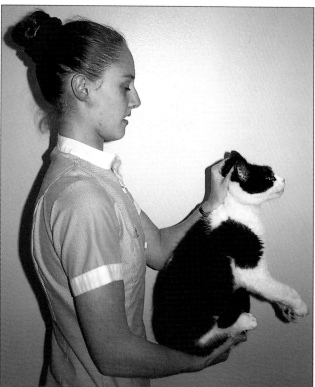

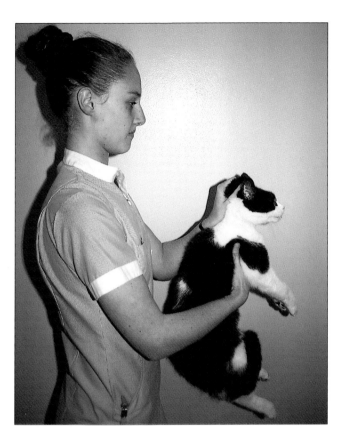

To carry a cat with a fractured hind limb or pelvis, hold the scruff of the neck and support the body under the chest.

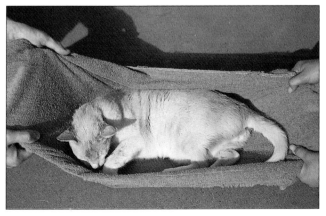

A towel can be used to make an improvised stretcher if a person stands at each end and takes a hold of the corners.

HOLDING

Hold the cat firmly by the scruff of the neck and the other hand around the chest and shoulders with the cat firmly held against your body.

• A cat may be held firmly in various ways according to the cat's problem and the treatment that has to be given.

• With the cat on a table:

- Hold the cat firmly by the scruff of the neck with one hand and cup the other hand around the chest and shoulders, holding the cat firmly against your body (see diagram).

- Or, hold the cat by the scruff of the neck with one hand

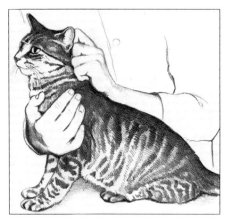

and place the other hand on the rump, at the same time applying downward pressure with both hands (see diagram).

- Or, stand behind the cat and lean over to hold the upper part of each foreleg in each of your hands. Your forearms and elbows should be pressed firmly against the cat's body.

- Or, if the cat is proving difficult to hold using these methods, wrap the cat securely in a blanket or large towel leaving exposed only that part of the body that requires attention (see diagram).

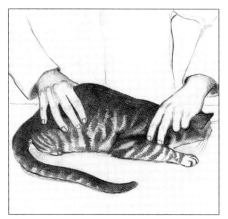

Hold the scruff of the neck with one hand and place the other hand on the rump, applying downward pressure with both hands.

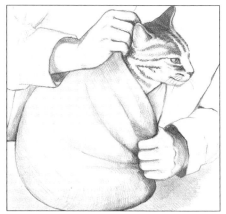

A good method of holding a difficult cat is to wrap it in a towel or blanket.

20

WHEN TO CALL YOUR VETERINARIAN

The following information may serve as a guide if you are uncertain when to call your veterinarian.

CALL IMMEDIATELY

• **Birth difficulty** No kitten appears after straining for 30 minutes; if, after straining for a period of time, the queen (mother) gives up; if part of a kitten appears but nothing else appears after 20 minutes of straining.

• **Bleeding heavily** From any part of the body; will not stop. Apply pressure to stop the bleeding on the way to the veterinarian (see page 58).

• **Blood in urine** Obvious blood in the urine.

• **Burns** Fairly extensive; or if in doubt.

• **Choking** Appears distressed; extends head and neck; salivates; coughs; paws at the mouth.

• **Collapse or loss of balance** Overreaction to external stimuli; depression; staggering or knuckling over; walking in circles; down and unable to get up; general muscle tremor; rigidity; paddling movements of legs; coma.

• **Pain** Severe, continuous or spasmodic.

• **Poisoning** Chemical, snake, spider or plant. If possible, retain sample for veterinarian to identify type of poisoning (see page 77).

• **Self-mutilation** Continual uncontrollable scratching, biting, tearing at the skin; skin broken and bleeding.

• **Severe breathing difficulty** Gasping; noisy breathing; blue tongue. If breathing not evident apply resuscitation (see page 44).

• **Severe injury** Severe continuous pain; severe lameness; cut with bone exposed; puncture wound, especially eye, chest or abdomen; fracture (see page 70); other injuries assessed as serious.

• **Straining continually** Attempting to defecate (pass a motion or stool) or urinate with little or no result.

• **Vomiting and/or severe diarrhea** Evidence of blood; putrid, fluid diarrhea.

CALL SAME DAY

• **Abortion (miscarriage)** Expulsion of the foetus after first three weeks of pregnancy.

• **Afterbirth** If retained for eight hours.

• **Appetite loss** Not eating; depressed in conjunction with other signs such as laboured breathing, diarrhea, lying down, pain.

• **Breathing difficulty** Laboured breathing; rapid and shallow breathing with or without cough.

• **Eye problems** Tears streaming down cheeks; eyelids partially or completely closed; cornea (surface of eye) cloudy, opaque or bluish-white in colour.

• **Frequent vomiting** Evident numerous occasions; associated with another symptom such as lethargy.

• **Frostbite and/or hypothermia** Low body temperature usually associated with sub-zero temperatures (see page 73 and/or 74).

• **Injury** Non-urgent but liable to become infected; a cut through full thickness of skin which needs stitching; puncture wound in leg or head; acute sudden lameness.

• **Mismating** Termination of an unwanted pregnancy can be done safely and harmlessly within 72 hours after intercourse.

• **Severe diarrhea** Motion (stool) fluid and putrid or there is abdominal pain or straining.

• **Severe itching** Biting; scratching; hair loss; skin red and inflamed.

• **Swallowed object** Better for veterinarian to assess early, rather than wait until a possible life-threatening situation develops.

• **Swelling** Hot, hard and painful or discharging.

WAIT 24 HOURS BEFORE CALLING

• **Appetite loss** Not eating; no other sign or symptom.

• **Diarrhea** Motion (stool) is semi-solid; no indication of abdominal pain; no sign of blood; no straining.

• **Itching** Moderate; no damage to the skin by self-mutilation.

• **Lameness** Ability to bear weight on leg; not affecting eating or other functions.

• **Occasional vomiting** On two or three occasions with no other symptoms.

• **Odour** Unpleasant odour other than a soiled coat.

• **Thirst** Excessive drinking, often paired with excessive urination.

TECHNIQUES YOU SHOULD KNOW

Bandaging

In serious, life-threatening situations, such as severe bleeding, it is important to apply firm pressure first, with the hand or a gauze pad and bandage, and clean the wound later.

Steps in bandaging

• If possible, clean the wound of any debris and clip any surrounding invasive hair. Cover the wound with a cotton gauze pad or a clean handkerchief.
• Wrap a cotton gauze bandage firmly over the pad covering the wound.
• Secure the gauze bandage by wrapping an adhesive bandage firmly over it, allowing some of the adhesive bandage to stick to the hair on either side of the gauze bandage.

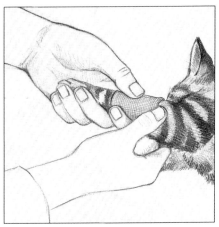

1. Cover the cleaned wound with a cotton gauze pad.

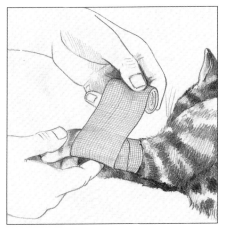

2. Wrap a cotton gauze bandage firmly over the pad.

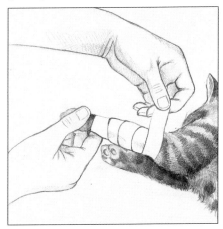

3. Secure the gauze bandage by firmly wrapping an adhesive bandage over it.

25

TYPES OF BANDAGE

Adhesive

• Provides a non-slip covering difficult for the cat to remove.
• Should never be applied directly to a wound except in an emergency.
• Ideal size is 2.5cm (1in) or 7.5cm (3in) wide.
• To avoid applying it too tightly, unroll a manageable portion first before wrapping it on.

Cotton gauze

• Gauze bandages alone tend to slip and are easily torn off by the cat.
• The best type is one that adheres to itself. It does not unravel and tends to conform to the shape of the cat, and it is firmer and not so bulky as a bandage.
• The end of the bandage can be secured by sticking it down with adhesive bandage. Another way is to cut the end down the middle to about 15cm (6in). Tie a knot at the base of the two tape-like pieces to prevent further tearing and tie the tapes to secure the bandage.
• The ideal size is 2.5cm (1in) wide.

Vetwrap bandage

• A strong, self-adhering bandage which will not unravel or slip and can be used more than once.
• It is soft and conforms to that part of the cat being bandaged.
• It is used to cover a gauze bandage or dressing.
• It is not as tough as an adhesive bandage and is more easily torn and pulled off by the cat.

HOW TO BANDAGE

Abdomen and chest

• Apply gauze pad after cleaning the wound.
• Fix pad with strips of adhesive bandage.
• Wrap cotton gauze bandage around the body four or five times.

• Apply adhesive bandage over the gauze bandage as well as the hair on either side.

Ear

• Clean the wound and cut away any invasive hair prior to bandaging.
• Place a gauze pad over the wound and secure it with adhesive strips.
• To stop the cat flicking or flapping the ear, lay the ear flat on top of the head and wrap a gauze bandage two to three times over that ear, under the neck and around behind the free ear. Secure with an adhesive bandage over it and the nearby hair. Carefully cut a small hole near the opening of the ear canal to allow air circulation to prevent any infection developing there.

Do you know?

• The cat's shape and coat of hair make it doubly difficult to apply a bandage that will stay in place.
• The most often bandaged areas are the abdomen, chest, ear, eye and limb.

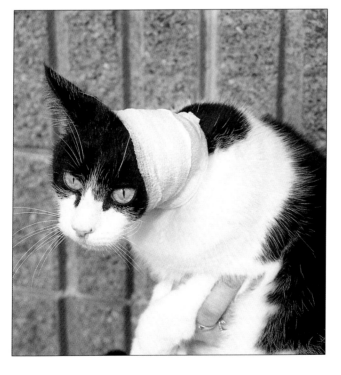

To stop a cat flicking an ear, lay the ear flat on top of the head and wrap a gauze bandage over that ear, under the neck and behind the free ear. Secure with an adhesive bandage.

27

Eye

• Apply gauze pad to the sore eye.
• Cover pad with a gauze bandage, starting behind the ear on the opposite side to the sore eye and passing it down across the sore eye, under the jaw and back behind the ear where it began. Repeat two to three turns of the bandage in this direction.
• Secure by wrapping an adhesive bandage over it and the nearby hair. If the cat tries to pull or rub the bandage off, apply an Elizabethan collar (see page 30).

Foot

• Clean the wound.
• Put cottonwool (absorbent cotton) between the toes.
• Apply a gauze pad to the wound.
• Wind gauze bandage around the paw, up beyond the largest pad, making it more secure by twisting it to face about after every two turns.
• Secure the bandage with adhesive bandage.

Leg

• Apply gauze pad to the wound after cleaning and cutting away any invasive hair.
• Wind cotton gauze bandage around the leg three to four times and secure with a similar adhesive bandage partly adhering to the cat's hair.

Keep in mind

• Bandages should never be too tight or too loose.
• If blood from a wound is coming through a bandage, do not remove but apply a slightly tighter adhesive bandage over it.
• If a very firm to tight bandage is on a limb for any length of time, for example, 30 minutes, check the limb below the bandage. If it is swollen, cold to the touch or does not react to pain when pinched, remove the bandage immediately and, if necessary, apply a new bandage less tightly.

Bleeding — How to Stop

- Remain calm.
- Immobilise the cat by holding firmly (see page 20).
- Apply pressure directly to the site with a clean wad of cloth or, if no cloth available, with your hand or fingers only.
- Apply an icepack to the site if the source of bleeding is inaccessible.
- The treatment required will vary according to the type and site of bleeding:
- Blood oozing slowly.
- Blood flowing freely.
- Blood spurting with a pulsating action.

See page 58 for further information on controlling these types of bleeding and page 25 for bandaging different body parts.

Caution

- Severe bleeding can be life threatening and should be controlled with First Aid treatment immediately and the cat taken to the veterinarian.
- Do not dab or wipe the site as this tends to promote bleeding.
- Do not clean the site until bleeding has stopped as this might encourage fresh bleeding.

Elizabethan collars will prevent a cat from interfering with a wound or injury.

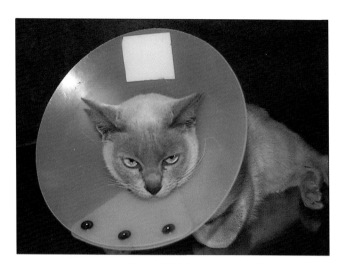

Elizabethan Collar — Making and Fitting

Wearing an Elizabethan collar prevents a cat licking itself, pulling out stitches, chewing a plaster cast, tearing off a bandage or scratching the ears or face. Your veterinarian can supply you with a commercial type or you can make your own, as follows:

• Select a suitably sized plastic bucket; that is, one in which, if you cut out the bottom, the head of the cat will just pass through. When it is in place the rim should protrude about 5cm (2in) beyond the cat's nose.
• Cut the appropriate-sized hole in the bottom of the bucket and punch six to ten evenly spaced small holes around the rim of the hole.
• Thread a short length of string or nylon cord through each small hole and tie each to make small loops so that the cat's collar can be passed through each one.
• Put the bucket over the cat's head and fasten the collar firmly so that the bucket is anchored to the cat's neck.

Caution

• Keep the cat confined or, if going for a walk, keep the cat on a lead as the Elizabethan collar limits the cat's field of vision.
• When the cat is to be fed, an alternative to taking off the collar is to hold the food or water bowl to the cat's mouth.

Heartbeat and Pulse — How to Check

The normal pulse of the cat varies according to breed, age and weight and ranges from 60 to 140 beats per minute.

• To obtain a correct reading, the cat must be calm.
• Place a finger (not the thumb) on the inside of the thigh near the groin and feel gently for a pulse from the artery just under the skin.

Where to Feel the Pulse

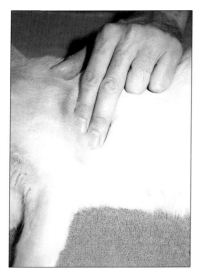
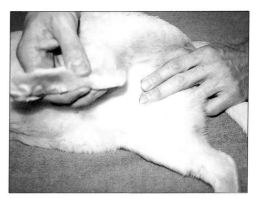

To feel the pulse place a finger on the inside of the thigh near the groin

The best place to feel the heartbeat is behind the left elbow between the third and sixth ribs.

31

**Where to Feel
the Heartbeat**

• The heartbeat is best located behind the left elbow between the third and sixth ribs.
• The beat can be observed as a regular slight movement of the chest wall on the left side in the area where the heart is located (see page 31).

**Heartbeat as a
Guide**

• If the heartbeat is an average 60 to 140 beats per minute, the circulation system is normal.
• If the heartbeat is outside the average range, see your veterinarian.

**No Heartbeat or
Pulse**

• Apply the cardiac compression technique immediately (see page 44).

Leg Fracture — Robert Jones Bandage Technique

The Robert Jones Bandage Technique described below (see also page 70) gives good immobilisation and support and does not interfere with circulation:

• Evenly wrap layers of cottonwool (absorbent cotton) around the fractured limb well above and below as well as over the apparent site of the fracture.
• Compress the layers of cottonwool by very firmly wrapping several rolls of gauze bandage over them.
• Finally, wrap a number of layers of adhesive bandage around the gauze bandage and nearby hair.
• Pinch the cat's toes to check that circulation has not been interfered with. If the cat reacts by pulling the foot away or crying, the pain sensation indicates good circulation.
• See page 34 for step-by-step photographs.

Medicine — How to Administer

Medicines come in many forms: tablet, capsule, powder, granule, liquid, paste, ointment, drops or injection. How the medicine is to be given and in what form depends on such factors as its type and palatability, the condition and temperament of the cat, and the owner's temperament. Some tablets, powders and granules are flavoured to make them palatable. This type can be handfed to the cat or mixed thoroughly with the cat's food. If it is mixed with the food, check the food bowl to make sure that the cat has eaten it. Cats are very suspicious of any foreign material in their food and some will sort it out or reject their food completely. If your cat's medicine is in the form of unpalatable tablets you can choose one of several methods to administer it: with your fingers; with a pill popper; or with a spoon. With each of these methods it is essential to know how to open a cat's mouth (see also page 35).

How to Open a Cat's Mouth

• Put the cat on a bench or table of suitable height in a small room, for example, the laundry.
• If the cat is restless, get someone to hold the cat firmly (see page 20) while you open the mouth in one quick movement.
• With one hand grasp the upper jaw between your fingers and thumb (see page 35).
• Tilt the cat's head back so that it is looking toward the ceiling; the mouth will open automatically.
• Using the middle finger of your other hand, press the front of the lower jaw down to open the mouth wider, but not too wide as the cat will become distressed.

Giving a Tablet with the Fingers

• Open the cat's mouth (see above) and place the tablet, held between the thumb and index finger, over the back of the cat's tongue. It may be necessary to quickly push the tablet further over the back of the tongue.

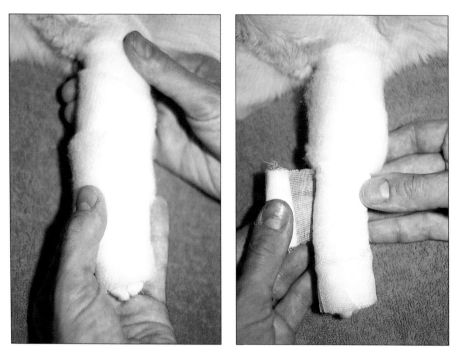

1. (top left) The Robert Jones Bandage Technique begins with wrapping layers of cottonwool (absorbent cotton) around the fractured limb.

2. (top right) Compress the cottonwool (absorbent cotton) by firmly wrapping several layers of gauze bandage over them.

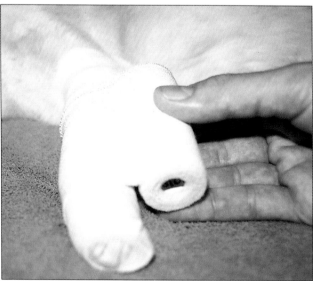

3. Finally, wrap layers of adhesive bandage around the gauze bandage and nearby hair.

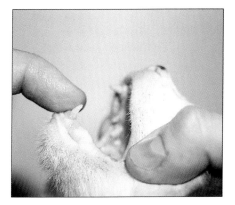

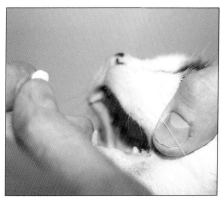

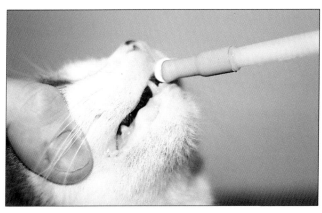

Top left: To open a cat's mouth, grasp the upper jaw and tilt the head back using the middle finger of your other hand to widen the opening.

Top right: Administering a tablet with the fingers.

Administering a tablet with a pill popper.

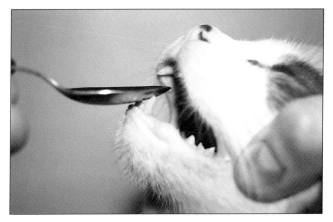

Administering a tablet with a spoon.

35

• Remove your finger quickly before the mouth closes.
• Keep the cat's head tilted back and massage the throat to stimulate swallowing. When the cat licks the upper lip with the tongue, the pill has been swallowed.

Caution

• Keep the cat's head tilted back or it will be difficult to drop the tablet over the back of the tongue.
• Ensure the tablet is over the back of the tongue or the cat will spit it out.

Giving a Tablet with a Pill Popper

• Put the tablet in the pill popper, a device used to place a tablet over the back of the cat's tongue.
• Open the cat's mouth (see pages 33 and 35).
• Quickly and smoothly place the end of the pill popper into the back of the cat's mouth.
• Press the plunger to release the tablet over the back of the tongue.
• Withdraw the popper, keep the cat's head tilted back and rub the throat to stimulate swallowing.

Giving a Tablet with a Spoon

• Place the tablet in a small spoon.
• Open the cat's mouth (see pages 33 and 35).
• Insert the spoon so that it is pressing down on the front of the lower jaw.
• Tip the tablet over the back of the tongue.
• Withdraw the spoon, keep the cat's head tilted back and rub the throat to stimulate swallowing.

Administering Liquids

• Open the cat's mouth with one hand and tilt the head back slightly (see pages 33 and 39).
• Holding a syringe or eye-dropper in the other hand, slowly dribble the liquid onto the back of the tongue.
• If the cat does not swallow, tilt the head a little more and dribble more liquid onto the back of the tongue.

Caution

• If the cat coughs and splutters, the liquid may be flowing into the windpipe. Correct by not tilting the head so far back.
• If the liquid is unpleasant, the cat may salivate profusely causing the liquid to dribble out of the mouth.
• Re-administer approximately the same amount of liquid as was dribbled. If concerned about a possible overdose, consult your veterinarian.

• Open the cat's mouth (see pages 33 and 38).
• Apply the paste, which usually comes in a syringe, to the cat's tongue. The paste will adhere to the tongue and be swallowed.
• Alternatively, mix the paste with the cat's favourite food; or smear the paste on the cat's forelimbs or around the mouth — the cat will lick the paste off.

Administering a Paste

Caution

• If the paste is unpalatable, the cat will salivate causing a mixture of paste and saliva to pour from the mouth.
• Re-administer approximately the same amount of paste as was dribbled. If concerned about a possible overdose, consult your veterinarian.

• Get an assistant to hold the cat firmly (see page 20) while you administer the ear drops.
• Take hold of the ear tip with your thumb and index finger, pulling it towards the opposite ear. This opens up the affected ear and makes the opening of the ear canal obvious.
• Squeeze four to six drops into the canal.
• Continue to hold the ear and the head firmly, otherwise the cat will shake the head vigorously and spray the drops everywhere (see page 39). If this happens, re-administer the same amount as was lost.

Administering Ear Drops

Paste can be administered directly onto the cat's tongue.

Alternately, paste can be smeared on the foreleg for the cat to lick.

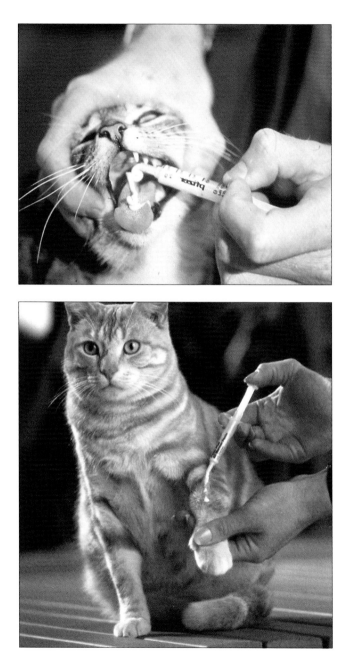

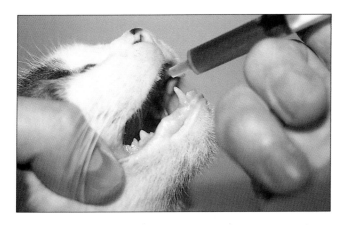

Administering liquid with a syringe.

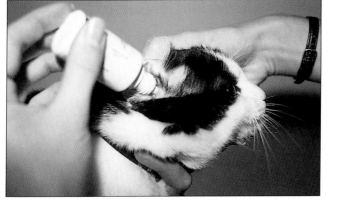

Adminstering drops into the ear canal.

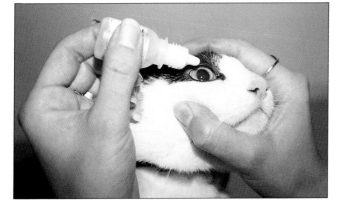

Keep the head tilted when administering eye drops.

• With your free hand gently massage below the ear to work the drops down the ear canal.
• If the cat is fidgety do not worry about counting the drops; just put the nozzle of the container in the ear canal and give it a squirt. Stop when you see the drops starting to well up out of the ear canal.

Administering Eye Drops

• Ask someone to hold the cat firmly (see page 20) and tilt the head back slightly.
• Gently hold the eyelids apart with your thumb and index finger.
• Administer two drops on each eyeball. Keep the head tilted for about 20 seconds or the eye drops will roll out and be wasted (see page 39).

Administering Eye Ointment

• Get an assistant to hold the cat firmly (see page 20) while you administer the medication.
• With your thumb, pull either the lower lid down or the upper lid up and lay a strip of eye ointment inside the lid along its full length.
• Close the eyelid. The ointment will melt forming a film over eyeball and conjunctiva.

Injections

If other methods of administering medicine are impossible because of the cat's temperament or condition, an injection may be the only alternative. This is best left to the veterinarian.

Orphan Kitten—How to Feed

Sometimes a kitten has to be handfed because the mother died at birth, or has no milk or rejects the kitten. Or, the kitten itself, because of weakness or for some other reason, is unable to suckle. When your kitten must be handfed, your veterinarian can supply you with a commercial milk substitute or you can make up your own using the formulas suggested below.

• Two formulas for substitute milk are:
- One cup of evaporated or powdered milk mixed with boiled water and made up to double the strength recommended on the container for babies. Mix in one egg yolk and one teaspoon of a glucose additive.
- Half a cup of cow's milk. Mix in one egg yolk and one teaspoon of a glucose additive.
• The faeces will give you an indication as to whether the milk substitute you are using is too rich. If the kitten has diarrhea, dilute the milk substitute. If diarrhea continues, consult your veterinarian.
• If possible, express the colostrum (first milk) from the mother's nipples and give it to the orphan kitten either with the substitute milk or separately.
• Warm the milk to body temperature before feeding.

Feeding Times

• Feed the kitten every two hours in the first week of life, giving about 5ml (1 teaspoon) of milk substitute at each feed. This amount can vary according to individual demand.
• Thereafter, gradually decrease the frequency of feeding and increase the amount of milk substitute.
• By the time the kitten is two weeks old, four-hourly feeding is sufficient.

Bottle Feeding

- Hold the kitten firmly, elevate the head slightly and insert the teat into the mouth.
- Move the teat in and out of the mouth and express a small amount of milk to encourage the kitten to suck.

Stomach Tube Feeding

- You will need a soft plastic tube 2mm (0.08in) in diameter and 15cm (6in) long, attached to a syringe.
- Measure the distance on the tube from the kitten's mouth to a point two-thirds along the rib cage.
- Mark the distance on the tube to indicate how far the tube has to be inserted via the kitten's mouth to reach the stomach.
- Insert the tube gently but firmly with great care, pushing it over the back of the tongue into the food pipe (esophagus), until it reaches the stomach.
- Ask your veterinarian to give you a demonstration or enlist the help of an experienced cat breeder.

Move the teat in and out when bottle feeding a kitten.

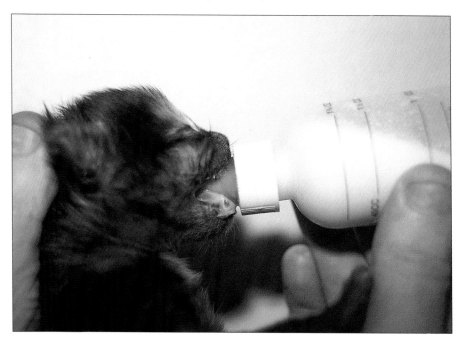

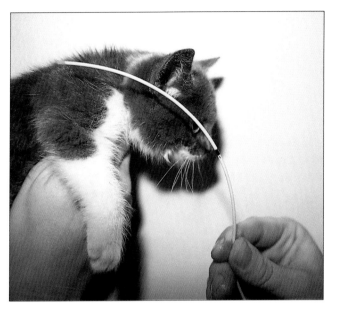

Measure a feeding tube from a kitten's mouth to a point two-thirds along the rib cage.

Insert the feeding tube gently but firmly.

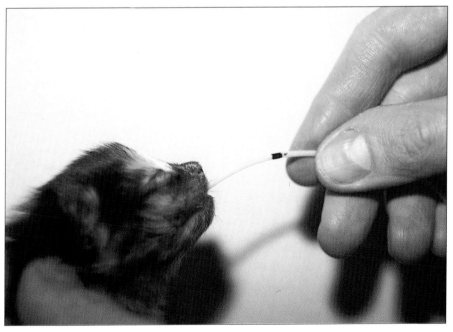

Resuscitation —
Breathing (Mouth-to-nose) and
Heartbeat (Cardiac Compression)

If Breathing has Stopped

• Check the cat's mouth or nose for any foreign body or food obstructing the airway. If an obstruction is present use one of the following methods to remove it:

- Hold the cat upside down by the hind legs and shake vigorously five or six times.
- Lay the cat on the side and, if necessary, use long-nosed pliers to clear any solid obstruction from the mouth.

• Lay the cat on the right side, tilt the head back and keep the mouth closed.
• Place a cloth, for example, a handkerchief, over the cat's nose (for cosmetic reasons).
• Place your open mouth over the cat's nose and quickly breathe into it five or six times. For a young kitten with a small lung capacity the breaths should be short and shallow; comparatively, for an adult cat the breaths should be longer and deeper, keeping in mind an adult cat has a relatively small lung capacity. The cat's mouth must be kept closed during the process (see page 46).
• If breathing is restored, keep the cat under observation.
• If breathing is not restored, apply mouth-to-nose resuscitation at the rate of one breath every two to three seconds; that is, 20 to 30 breaths per minute.
• Continue until breathing is restored. If it is, keep the cat under observation.
• If breathing is not restored after 10 minutes, if the gums and tongue are blue, the pupils are dilated and there is no blinking when the surface of the eye is touched, you can presume that the cat is dead.

Do you know?

• The average cat's breathing rate is 20 to 30 breaths per minute.
• The average cat's heartbeat (pulse rate) is 60 to 140 per minute.
• Immediate, yet calm, treatment is essential in resuscitation.

• Lay the cat on the right side.
• If a kitten, with one hand place your thumb on one side of the chest and your fingers on the other in the area between the third and sixth ribs just behind the left elbow.
• If an adult cat, place fingers as shown in the photograph (see page 46) over the area between the third and sixth ribs just behind the left elbow.
• The force applied to the heart area in cardiac compression varies according to the size of the cat, from light fingertip compression for a young kitten to moderate fingertip compression for an adult cat.
• Give 10 quick compressions. If the heartbeat and pulse are restored, keep the cat under observation.
• If the heartbeat and pulse are not restored, continue to apply cardiac compression in cycles of 10 at the rate of 10 cycles per minute, that is about one cycle every six seconds. When the heartbeat and pulse are restored, keep the cat under observation.
• If there is no sign of heartbeat and pulse after 10 minutes, if the gums and tongue are blue, the pupils are dilated and there is no blinking when the surface of the eye is touched, you can presume that the cat is dead.

If Heartbeat (Pulse) has Stopped

• If there are two people present: one person gives about 10 cardiac compressions followed by the second person giving two mouth-to-nose expired air breaths. Repeat this synchronised sequence at the rate of about 10 cycles per minute, that is about one sequence every six seconds.
• If only one person is present: give 10 cardiac compressions followed by two mouth-to-nose expired air breaths. Repeat this sequence at the rate of about 10 cycles per minute, that is about one sequence every six seconds.
• See the section above for signs to check after 10 minutes.

If Breathing and Heartbeat (Pulse) have Stopped

To resuscitate a cat, keep the cat's mouth closed, place your open mouth over the cat's nose, covered with a cloth, and quickly breathe into it.

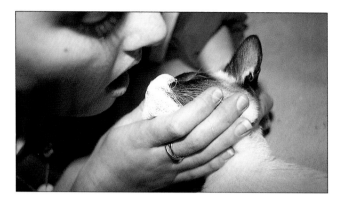

Fingers should be placed in this position when giving cardiac massage to an adult cat.

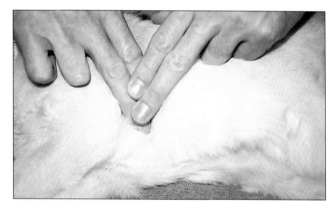

Temperature — How to Check

• The normal temperature for a cat ranges between 37.8°C (100°F) and 39.2°C (102.5°F).
• If your cat's temperature remains outside that range see your veterinarian, as the cat probably has an infection or some other illness.

Action

• An ordinary household thermometer may be used.
• Shake the mercury down to below 37.8°C (100°F) and smear the thermometer with a non-irritant lubricant, such as Vaseline.

46

- Insert the thermometer into the cat's anus to about 5cm (2in), with the bulb resting against the rectal wall.
- Withdraw the thermometer after one to two minutes and check the reading.
- Clean the thermometer with disinfectant and store in a suitable container.
- Wash your hands thoroughly.

Umbilical Cord — How to Sever and Treat

- The queen (mother) often breaks the umbilical cord when she is licking, pulling and tearing at the foetal membrane to free the kitten.
- If the umbilical cord is not broken, wait five to 10 minutes before severing it; otherwise, the kitten may suffer brain damage.

Action

- To prevent bleeding, apply a ligature by tightly tying thread soaked in disinfectant around the umbilical cord about 2cm (3/4in) from the kitten's body.
- Cut the cord with scissors soaked in disinfectant 1cm (1/3in) from the ligature, on the placental side. Or, break the cord with your fingers.
- Swab the cut end with tincture of iodine.

Caution

- Premature breaking of the cord may deprive the kitten of its maximum blood supply, thus starving the brain of oxygen causing subsequent damage.
- If the end of the cord is bleeding when severed by the queen, control the hemorrhage by tying the cord off with disinfected thread.

FIRST AID FOR INJURIES AND ILLNESS

Abscess

Causes

- Abscesses in most cases are caused by fighting with another cat. When a tooth or claw penetrates the skin it causes damage to underlying tissue. Bacteria are deposited in the tissue at the time of penetration.
- Foreign bodies, such as a splinter of wood or a grass seed, are not a common cause of abscesses in cats.

Signs

- An abscess is a collection of pus, circumscribed in a sac, and enclosed within the tissues of the body.
- Pain is felt by the cat when touched at the site of the abscess.
- The cat may be lethargic, without an appetite and/or have a temperature.
- The abscess is at first a hard lump which softens as it matures and finally may burst
- Puncture wounds from a bite or a sharp foreign body are common causes.

Action

- Cut away surrounding hair and bathe the wound with a cloth or cottonwool (absorbent cotton) soaked in hot water for 10 minutes twice daily.
- If a puncture wound is obvious, clean with iodine-based scrub or 3% hydrogen peroxide. Remove any foreign body that may be embedded in the wound.
- If the abscess bursts, clean as suggested and gently squeeze out any evident discharge.
- If the abscess does not burst, the veterinarian will open the abscess, drain out the pus and administer antibiotics.
- If the abscess continues to drain after being opened, it should be irrigated twice daily using a syringe containing 3% hydrogen peroxide.

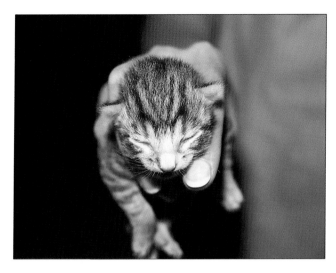

This grip should be used with one form of resuscitation for newborn kittens. Cradle the kitten in your hand with the head protruding between your index and middle fingers. See page 53.

Birth Problems

• Kittens are usually born 10 to 30 minutes apart.
• All the kittens are usually born over a period of three to six hours.
• The normal presentation of the newborn kitten at the vulva is head first.
• If the kitten is born in its amnion sac (membrane), the queen ruptures it with her teeth to release the kitten, licks the kitten to clean it and chews through the umbilical cord if it is not broken. If the queen neglects to do so, you must do it, especially cleaning the kitten's airways (nose and mouth) of any membrane and mucus so that it can breathe. See page 47 for breaking of the umbilical cord.
• In rendering First Aid at a birth scene make sure that your hands have been scrubbed with a non-irritant antiseptic and that you are wearing surgical gloves if available.
• If you cannot give the necessary First Aid, get in touch with your veterinarian immediately.

Signs

Kitten's head presented at the vulva, but the queen (mother) cannot expel it

• Scrub your hands and clean the area around the queen's anus and vulva with a non-irritant antiseptic.
• If the membranes are intact, break them with your fingers to clear the kitten's nose and mouth so that breathing is possible.
• Prepare to get a good grip of the kitten by removing any visible membrane and, with a piece of clean towelling material in your hand, take hold of the kitten around the shoulder area.
• Slowly pull outward and downward. If the kitten will not budge, a twist to the left or right in conjunction with pulling will often bring about success.

One leg presented at the vulva

• Put your finger into the vagina and feel for the other leg. Gently pull it outward, then proceed to deliver the kitten.

Hindquarters presented at the vulva

• Take hold of the kitten in the region of the hips. Pull outward and downward.

Caution

• Avoid squeezing the abdomen as this can cause serious damage.

No kitten present at the vulva

• Call your veterinarian if:

- The queen (mother) has been straining for more than 30 minutes and no kitten appears.
- There are no obvious contractions and the queen is distressed, continually getting up and down, looking at her flanks and crying.

- After 30 minutes of obvious straining and contractions, the queen appears to give up and her efforts are weak and less frequent.

Newborn kitten not breathing

• Check pulse and heartbeat (see page 31).
• Check the airways to see that they are clear. If necessary, wipe away any placental membranes or mucus that may be blocking the kitten's nostrils or mouth.
• Lay the kitten, with the head lower than the rest of the body, on a towel wrapped around a hot water bottle (not too hot). Warmth is very important and the head-down position allows blood to flow more freely to the brain.
• Rub the kitten's chest briskly with a towel to stimulate breathing.
• If the kitten is still not breathing gently massage the chest, positioned between your thumb and fingers.
• If still no sign of breathing, grip the kitten safely cradled in your hand with the head protruding from between your index and middle fingers (see page 51). Raise the held kitten above your head and proceed with an action as if you were going to throw the kitten to the ground. Repeat this action four or five times to rid the nose and mouth of any mucus and stimulate respiration.
• Finally, if the kitten is still not breathing, apply mouth-to-nose resuscitation (see page 44). A newborn kitten has only a small lung capacity so use short, shallow breaths to avoid stretching or rupturing the lungs.

Afterbirth not expelled

Afterbirth is normally expelled with the birth of each kitten or immediately after. Often the queen (mother) will eat the afterbirth, so it may not be seen. If the afterbirth(s) is (are) not expelled within eight hours after the last kitten is born, take the following action:

• If the retained afterbirth is obvious, remove it by manually pulling on it with firm, even tension.
• If this fails or the retained afterbirth is not obvious, *contact your veterinarian.*

Bites and Stings

CAT BITE

Cats inflict puncture wounds with their canine teeth and claws when fighting.

Signs

• A painful spot and/or blood matted in the hair.
• The usual site of puncture wounds is the head, forelimbs, back, or base of tail.
• A puncture wound may look neat and clean on the surface, but tissue under the skin can be badly torn and infected.

Action

• Carefully clip the hair away from the wound.
• Clean the area with 3% hydrogen peroxide and dab the wound with tincture of iodine.
• If the puncture wound appears to penetrate through the skin into the underlying tissue, take the cat to the veterinarian who will administer antibiotics and, if necessary, drain the wound.

Caution

• Some types of puncture wound may lead to an abscess (see page 50) or serious infection.

TICK BITE
Signs

• An early sign is a change in the cat's voice to a croaky, husky meow.
• If the tick is about the cat's face, it may cause paralysis of eyelids or lip on the side that the tick is located.
• Pupils are dilated. The tongue may poke out of the mouth and the cat may vomit.

• Paralysis progresses to hind limbs and chest, when a further sign will be grunting, distressed breathing.
• Paralysis of chest muscles leads to death by suffocation.

Action

• Hold the hair away from the tick so that you can see where the head is embedded in the skin.
• Grasp the tick with tweezers as close to its embedded head as possible and pull it out.
• If part of the head is left in the skin do not worry, but dab with antiseptic.

Caution

• If at any time the cat shows sign(s) of tick poisoning, take the cat to the veterinarian for anti-tick serum and observation.

Do you know?

• Only the adult female tick attaches itself to the cat and in four to six days will poison it, eventually causing paralysis and death.
• The adult female tick, oval in shape, varies in colour from grey to blue to brown. It varies in size from 2mm (⅛in) to 8mm (⅓in) depending on its engorgement with blood.

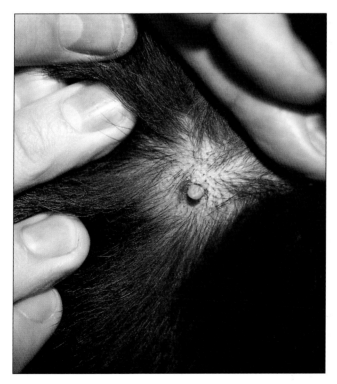

Hold hair away from the tick to reveal where the head is embedded.

Prevention

• Ticks are active in late spring and early summer and it is best to keep the cat away from heavy plant growth and long grass at this time. Cats should be checked for ticks daily during this period.
• Keep in mind that 80 per cent of ticks found are on the cat's head and neck; the remaining 20 per cent are on any other part of the cat.
• Rinse the cat each week with an insecticidal solution.
• Clip long-haired cats in spring. Ticks do not attach themselves as readily to short-haired cats and are easier to find.

SNAKE BITE
Signs

• The cat is stunned, often slobbering from the mouth.
• The cat has staring, unblinking eyes.
• There is little limb movement.
• The cat may be lying on the side or chest.
• You can tell whether your cat has been bitten by a poisonous or a non-poisonous snake by the bite mark. Poisonous snakes leave two fang marks (puncture wounds); the non-poisonous ones leave a row of small teeth marks.
• As usually you do not see your cat being bitten by a snake, knowing the signs is important.

Action

If the cat has been bitten on a leg

• Calm the cat (see page 14).
• Apply a broad bandage with firm pressure over the fang marks and about 5cm (2in) either side of them.

If the cat has been bitten in an area that is difficult to bandage

• Calm the cat (see page 14).
• Apply an icepack (for example, ice in a towel) to the site to constrict blood vessels.
• Seek veterinary help immediately. If you did see the

> **Do you know?**
> • Snake bites are less of a problem in the UK where there is only one poisonous snake —the adder.

snake, keep a good description of it in mind, as the veterinarian will choose from several different types of antivenene (anti-venom) in treating your cat.

Caution

• *Do not* apply a tourniquet as it may aggravate the problem.
• *Do not* cut the skin at the bite site as it will increase blood flow and spread of the poison.

The active cat, searching about in the garden with its nose and forelimbs, may be bitten or stung by an insect such as a bee, by a spider, or by some plant to which it is allergic.

UNIDENTIFIED BITE OR STING

Signs will vary but may include:

• Sudden pain and crying.
• Rapid swelling or welts on face or paw, perhaps with inflammation.
• The cat scratching or biting the affected area.

Signs

Check the site where the incident occurred. It may help you to find the cause, and:

• If a bee, remove the sting and apply a cold compress or soothing lotion, for example, calamine.
• If a spider, identify it and if poisonous take the cat to your veterinarian.
• If swelling is extensive, or the cat appears distressed or in a state of shock (see page 86), seek veterinary advice.

Action

Do you know?

• There are no poisonous spiders in the UK.

Bleeding

To control the cat's bleeding

- Remain calm.
- Immobilise the cat by holding firmly (see page 20).
- Apply pressure directly to the site or apply an icepack (for example, ice in a towel) if the site is inaccessible.
- Apply a bandage firmly to the site (see page 25).

Caution

- Do not dab, wipe or attempt to clean the site until after the bleeding stops as each tends to promote bleeding.

If blood is oozing slowly

- Place a clean gauze pad on the wound and apply direct pressure on it with your fingers.
- After 10 seconds, remove the gauze pad to evaluate the wound
- If bleeding recommences, reapply gauze pad and finger pressure for a longer time, about 20 seconds.

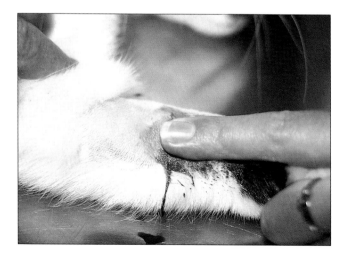

Apply pressure directly to the site of bleeding.

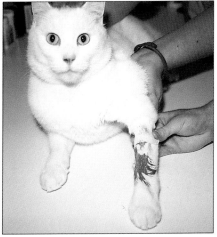

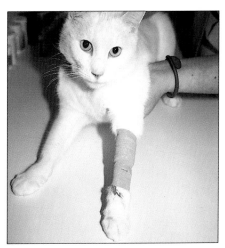

1. To stop bleeding place a clean gauze pad on the wound and apply pressure.

2. Wrap an adhesive bandage firmly but not too tightly over the gauze pad.

If blood is flowing freely

• Place a gauze pad on the wound and apply heavy, direct pressure with clean fingers or hand for about 30 seconds.
• Over the gauze pad wrap firmly but not too tightly a 7.5cm (3in) wide adhesive bandage;
• Leave the bandage in place for 30 minutes, then remove it to evaluate the wound;
• If bleeding recommences, reapply the pressure bandage.

If the blood is bright red, spurting with pulsating action

• This is a sign of arterial bleeding.
• With a gauze pad in hand, apply heavy pressure to the site for about 30 seconds.
• Wrap a 7.5cm (3in) adhesive bandage tightly around the gauze pad
• Leave the bandage in place, keep the cat immobilised, preferably wrapped in a blanket (see page 20), and take

the cat to your veterinarian
• If blood is oozing or running through the bandage, do not remove it but apply another adhesive bandage more tightly over the top of it.

If blood is coming from an inaccessible area, for example, inside the nose

• Apply cold in the form of an icepack and keep the cat immobilised (see page 20).

Caution

• The cat may bleed to death if you panic and hesitate.
• Keep the cat still, as movement will accelerate the bleeding. The ideal is for one person to immobilise the cat while another person controls the bleeding (see page 20).
• When a pressure bandage is left on a limb for 30 minutes, always check the limb below the bandage for swelling, coldness, or non-reaction to pain if pinched. If any of these signs is evident, release the bandage and reapply it less firmly.
• Tourniquets are not recommended. They are often difficult to apply and if applied incorrectly, may accentuate rather than retard bleeding.
• Take the cat to the veterinarian as soon as the bleeding is under control.

Burns

CHEMICAL BURN

Many household products such as chlorine can cause burns, mostly to the skin and sometimes internally.

Action

• If on skin, wash thoroughly by hosing or pouring copious amounts of water on the cat for about five

minutes, then gently wash the area with soap and water. Rinse thoroughly.
• If ingested, encourage the cat to drink copious amounts of water. If the cat refuses, use a syringe or gently running water from the hose to rinse the cat's mouth, thereby stimulating drinking. In the case of acid burn use sodium bicarbonate solution (baking soda) as an alternative, to neutralise the acid.
• Take the cat to your veterinarian.

ELECTRICAL BURN

The main risk is kittens or playful cats biting a moving electrical lead attached to, for instance, an iron or lawn mower. A blow-drier falling into the bathtub while the cat is being washed also presents a danger.

Action

• Turn the power off at the switch.
• If unable to get to the switch, use a dry wooden or plastic stick to flick the plug out of the socket and to push the cat away from the source of electricity.
• Check the cat's breathing and heartbeat (see page 31). If necessary, apply resuscitation (see page 44).
• Take the cat to your veterinarian.

HEAT BURN
Signs

• First-degree burns are the least serious; signs are various degrees of reddened skin.
• Second-degree burns are characterised by reddening of the skin with the formation of blisters.
• Third-degree burns are the most serious and are characterised by the full thickness of the skin and underlying tissue being destroyed.
• Extensive second- and third-degree burns are associated with shock, fluid loss (dehydration) and infection.
• The burn may be fatal if more than 50 per cent of the cat's skin is affected.

Action

- Immediately run cold water on the burn from a hose, tap or shower; or, if ice is readily available, apply it for 10 to 15 minutes; or immerse the burnt area in a basin filled with water and ice.
- Dry the area by dabbing gently. Do not rub as you may break the delicate surface.
- In the case of a second- or third-degree burn, protect the wound by covering it gently with a gauze pad or clean handkerchief held in place with a light adhesive bandage. Do not use cottonwool (absorbent cotton) because it will adhere to the surface of the burn.
- Deep or extensive burns require quick veterinary attention.

Choking

Signs

- Attempting to vomit.
- Mouth open and the cat does not appear able to close it.
- Saliva dribbling from the mouth.
- Clawing of the mouth with the front paws.
- If breathing reasonably freely, take the cat to your veterinarian immediately.

Action

- If the cat is on the verge of collapsing and the tongue is blue:
- Wedge something, such as the handle of a small screwdriver, between the molar teeth on one side of the cat's mouth to keep it open.
- Inspect the back of the throat, roof of the mouth and between the teeth for a foreign body.
- Pull the tongue out carefully to avoid being bitten — a foreign body over the back of the tongue may be found.
- Use long-nosed pliers or, if the mouth of the cat cannot close, use your finger(s) to lever the foreign body out.
- If you are unable to remove the foreign body by the above method, hold the cat upside down by the hind

legs. Shake the cat vigorously to dislodge the foreign body and clear the airway.

• If the cat is not breathing (see page 31), give mouth-to-nose resuscitation (see page 44).

Conjunctivitis

• The conjunctiva is the membrane lining the inside of the eyelids.
• Conjunctivitis is inflammation and/or infection of the conjunctiva.
• Kittens' eyes open seven to ten days after birth. If an infection of the conjunctiva is present it is usually noticed at that time.

Signs

• The cat's eyelids are stuck together.
• Pus oozes from the corner of the eyelids.
• Dry pus adheres to the edges of the eyelids.

Action

• Bathe the eyelids in warm water and gently part them; be careful not to pull the eyelids apart too abruptly because you may damage the rims.
• Wipe away any discharge adhering to the eyelashes or eyelids while bathing them. This helps to prevent them sealing together again.
• Keep the cat out of the wind and direct sunlight.
• If the discharge from the cat's eye is heavy or continuous, see your veterinarian who will prescribe an appropriate eye ointment.

Caution

• There are numerous eye ointments, each of which has a specific purpose. Eye ointments should not be used indiscriminately for conjunctivitis as the wrong kind can worsen certain conditions. For example, if an ulceration of the cornea (the surface of the eyeball) is incorrectly treated the result may be blindness or an otherwise damaged eye.

Diabetic Emergency *(Insulin Overdose)*

An overdose of insulin causes hypoglycaemia — that is, a low blood sugar level — that can result in convulsions, coma and possibly death.

Action for Low Blood Sugar Level Due to Insulin Overdose

• If the cat is conscious but not coordinated enough to be able to eat, use a syringe to carefully give through the mouth large amounts of sugar dissolved in water, or honey, maple syrup, etc.
• If the cat can eat, give canned or dried food, or cakes, biscuits or any food high in sugar.
• *Seek veterinary help.*
• Once the condition is stabilised, the veterinarian will supply you with sticks to test the urine sugar level, and needles, syringes and insulin to maintain the correct level.

Diarrhea

Signs

• The cat defecates more frequently, and the faeces are of a porridge or fluid-like consistency, often with a very offensive odour.

Action

• Do not feed the cat for 24 hours but provide drinking water.
• If the cat has not passed a motion (stool) or the motion appears firmer, offer a small amount (a quarter of normal daily food intake) of steamed chicken or lean, grilled meat.

• Exclude dairy products and fat from the diet until the cat has fully recovered.
• After three to four days of normal motions, slowly return the cat to a normal diet.
• If the diarrhea persists for more than 24 hours, there is blood in the motion, the cat is lethargic, vomits, or appears to have a loss of appetite, take the cat and a specimen of the faeces to your veterinarian for examination.

Drowning

Very young, very old and sick or injured cats are more likely to drown although healthy, fit cats sometimes drown following fatigue if they are unable to get out of the water.

Action

• Quickly remove the cat from the water.
• If breathing, hold the cat upside down by the hind legs. After a short time, place the cat in a position where the head is lower than the chest. This action helps to drain water from the lungs.
• If the cat's breathing or heart (pulse) has stopped (see page 31), apply resuscitation (see page 44).

Prevention

• If you or your neighbour have a swimming pool make sure that the cat knows how and where to get out of it.

Ear Haematoma

Signs

• Ear haematoma is a circumscribed swelling of the ear flap containing blood. It is usually caused by the cat scratching and shaking the ear, or by a blow or bite from another cat that ruptures a blood vessel in the ear flap.

Action

• When the blood vessel in the ear flap first breaks, apply an icepack for 10 to 15 minutes to stop the bleeding and reduce the swelling.
• If the swelling is small, apply pressure for 10 to 15 minutes with your thumb on one side of the ear flap and your index finger on the other side.
• If the haematoma persists, take your cat to the veterinarian who will anaesthetise the cat and drain the haematoma. If the haematoma is not drained, the blood forms into a hard, fibrous swelling, distorting the shape of the ear—like the cauliflower ear seen in humans.

Eye Injuries

• Any injury to the eyeball or eyelids should be regarded as serious.
• Damage to the eyeball may lead to permanent blindness.
• Any break in an eyelid may lead to tear loss and a dry eye.

Action

• Place a wad of cottonwool (absorbent cotton) soaked in water over the eye to keep eyelids and/or eyeball moist.
• Seek veterinary attention immediately.

EYEBALL PROLAPSE (EYE POPPED OUT OF THE SOCKET) Action

• Keep the eyeball moist with a cottonwool (absorbent cotton) ball soaked in water.
• Attempt to pull the eyelids over the protruding eyeball. If successful, apply firm, even pressure to push (not force) the eyeball back into the socket.
• Seek veterinary attention immediately.

CHLORINE OR CEMENT BURNS TO EYE

Because the eye is moist, chlorine or cement will adhere to the eye, burning it and in some cases causing permanent damage or blindness.

Action

• Wash the eye immediately and repeatedly, using such techniques as:

66

- A syringe filled with clean water.
- A very gentle stream of water from a hose.
- Wiping the eye gently until clean with a cottonwool (absorbent cotton) ball saturated in water, then dripping water onto the eye from a saturated cottonwool ball.
• Seek veterinary help quickly.

Foreign bodies such as a grass seed can cause permanent damage to the eye.

FOREIGN BODY IN EYE

Action

• Wash the eye with copious amounts of water.
• Gently open and close the eyelids to work the foreign body toward the corner of the eyelids or to make it visible.
• If visible, carefully attempt to remove the foreign body.
• If unable to remove, or if after removal the cat is very uncomfortable, seek veterinary assistance.
• Seek veterinary assistance if cat's eye is tightly closed and you cannot identify the problem.

Fishhook Caught in Lip

If the cat is quiet and the barbed end of the hook is protruding through the lip

• With an assistant holding the cat's head very firmly to keep it still (see page 20), cut through the hook with a pair of pliers or metal cutters at a point between the barb and the skin, or between the eye of the hook and the skin, whichever is the more convenient.
• The remainder of the hook can then be removed.

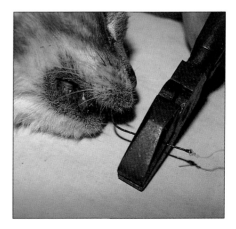

If the cat is agitated or the barbed end of the hook is embedded in the lip or mouth

• Seek veterinary assistance.

Caution

• Do not push or pull the hook.

Fishing Line or Thread Disappearing into Mouth

Caution

• Do not cut the line or thread. It may be attached to a fishhook or needle and could be of use to the veterinarian in locating and removing either of these objects.

Action

• Open the cat's mouth.
• If the fishing line or cotton disappears over the back of the tongue, gently pull the line or thread.
• If it will not budge, do not persist in pulling.
• Seek veterinary help.

Fit or Convulsion

A fit usually lasts for a minute or two, then the cat recovers.

Signs

• Lying on side.
• Unconscious.
• Paddling of legs.
• Champing of jaws.
• Frothing at mouth.
• Twitching.

Caution

• Do not try to take hold of the cat's tongue as you may be badly bitten by the champing jaws of the unconscious cat.

Action

• Observe the cat but do not touch. Touching may prolong and aggravate the seizure.
• Once recovered, the cat may seem a little disorientated. Make an appointment to see your veterinarian.
• If the cat continues fitting beyond five minutes, take the cat to your veterinarian immediately.
• If the cat is taking a series of fits, in between fits lift the cat gently into the car and go immediately to your veterinarian. (See page 14 for handling an injured cat).
• If the cat is impossible to handle, call your veterinarian for help.

Foreign Body in Ear

Cats with ears covered with long hair are more susceptible to foreign bodies, the most common being grass seed.

Signs

• Shaking the head vigorously, frequently holding the head to one side and scratching the affected ear.

Action

• Check the ear flap inside and out.
• Ask an assistant to hold the cat's head still (see page 20).
• Use a torch to examine the ear canal and, if discharge is present, clean it out with a cotton bud (swab). If a foreign body is present it usually comes away with the discharge. If the foreign body remains embedded, remove it with blunt-ended tweezers.
• If you are unable to locate or remove a foreign body and the cat is distressed, see your veterinarian.

Use blunt-ended tweezers (forceps) to remove a foreign body from the ear.

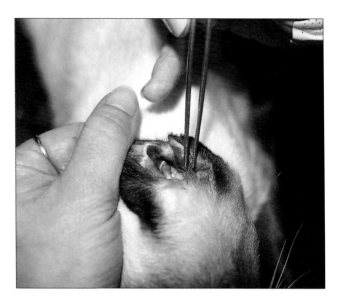

Fracture

Types of fracture

• **Clean break** A simple clean break.

• **Greenstick** Generally a bone fracture of young cats in which one side of the bone is broken and the opposite side is intact.

• **Hairline** A crack indicated by a fine line which may not go through the full thickness of the bone.

• **Impacted** One fractured end of the bone is forced into the other.

• **Multiple** The bone is broken in two or more places.

• **Compound** The fractured end of the bone protrudes through the skin. This is a serious fracture because of the danger of infection. Cover the wound with a gauze swab or a clean linen cloth, for example, a handkerchief, then apply a bandage using the Robert Jones technique as described for a leg fracture (see page 32 and 71).

> **Do you know?**
>
> The majority of fractures in the cat involve the limbs, pelvis, lower jaw or spine.

70

• A fracture causes pain. A cat in pain may bite, so take special care in handling or moving a cat that might have a fracture (see page 14).
• If the injured cat is in a danger zone, for example, a busy street, move it carefully to a safe area before applying First Aid.
• In giving First Aid your aim is to prevent the fracture and surrounding injured area from being worsened, especially during transit to the veterinary hospital.

Signs

• Swelling.
• Pain.
• Holding a limb off the ground.
• Limb(s) misshapen or dangling.
• Both hind legs are collapsed.
• Cat unable to move hind legs or all four limbs.

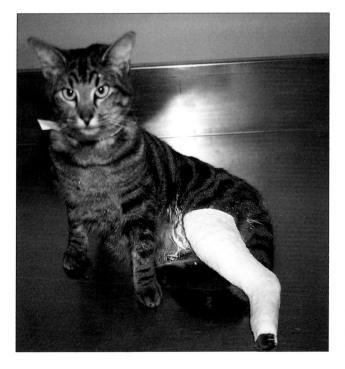

A plaster cast has been applied by a veterinarian on this fractured hind leg.

71

Action

For a leg fracture

• Apply a bandage using the Robert Jones technique: evenly wrap layers of cottonwool (absorbent cotton) around the leg, well above and below as well as over the site of the fracture. Very firmly wrap gauze bandage over the cottonwool, compressing it, then cover the bandage and nearby hair with an adhesive bandage (see page 32).

• Lift and carry the cat to your car, for transit to the veterinarian. If a forelimb is fractured, pick up the cat by the scruff of the neck in one hand and support the body by capping your other hand around the hindquarters. If a hind limb is fractured, pick up the cat by the scruff of the neck with one hand and support the body by placing your other hand under the chest (see page 18 and 19).

For a spine fracture

• If the cat cannot use the hind legs and there is no reaction when you pinch the toes, suspect a middle to lower spine fracture.

• If the cat cannot use the forelegs and hind legs, suspect a neck injury.

• *Very carefully* pull the cat on to a towel or folded blanket placed alongside. With one person at each end to hold the corners, the blanket or towel can be used as a stretcher. Take the cat to your veterinarian (see page 19).

Caution

• Transport the cat with minimal movement of the spine to prevent any further damage to the spinal cord.

For a pelvic fracture

• If the cat is unable to stand on the hind legs, there is a possible multiple fracture of the pelvis.

• If the cat is able to walk tentatively with the hind legs, there is a possible minor fracture.

• Pick up the cat by the scruff of the neck with one hand

and support the body by placing your other hand under the chest (see page 19).

• Take the cat to your veterinarian.

For a jaw fracture

• Generally, fracture of the jaw does not require immobilisation.
• Take the cat to your veterinarian.

Frostbite

Signs

• The skin is pale white in colour, has no sensation and is very cold to the touch.

Action

• If wet, dry the cat thoroughly.
• Wrap the cat in a thick, warm blanket.
• Warm the frostbitten area in a bath at approximately 40°C (104°F) for about 10 minutes.
• Apply a pad soaked in the same warm water (40°C or 104°F) to areas such as the tips of the ears.
• If the circulation returns, the skin will become red, swollen and look like a burn.
• Depending on the depth of the frostbite, if the circulation does not return the skin will peel or a demarcation line will develop between the live and dead tissue.
• If only the superficial skin layers are peeling, apply a soothing antibiotic cream to soften the skin and control infection.
• If the tissues are pale, cold and insensitive after warming for 20 minutes, *see your veterinarian.*

Do you know?

• Cats exposed to temperatures below freezing point for lengthy periods are susceptible to frostbite.
• Cats with short hair are more susceptible than others.
• The ears, toes and tail—are the sites most often affected.

73

Heatstroke

• Prolonged heatstroke can lead to coma, brain damage or death.
• Cats have no sweat glands and only regulate their body temperature by panting.

Signs

• Panting.
• Mouth open, gasping for air.
• Distressed.
• Often unable to stand.
• Movement uncontrolled and agitated.
• Gums are deep red.

Action

• Cool the cat immediately by wetting thoroughly with cold water, placing in front of a fan or in a cool, shady area with easy access to water as the cat improves.
• Seek veterinary help if the cat does not respond to treatment after 10 minutes.

Prevention

• Do not leave your cat confined in a poorly ventilated area in hot weather, for example, in a car with all the windows closed.
• Ensure that the cat has access to cool water and a cool, shady area in very hot weather.

Do you know?

• Cats are inefficient at getting rid of body heat, especially in hot weather, but efficient at retaining body heat in cold weather.

Hypothermia (Low Body Temperature)

Hypothermia is most often observed in newborn kittens because they are unable to regulate their body temperature. A fullgrown healthy cat subjected to cold conditions normally does not suffer from hypothermia.

However, keep in mind that the breed of cat and length of exposure to a certain temperature will have a bearing on whether or not the cat will suffer from hypothermia.

Signs

- Initially the kitten is restless, constantly crying and cold to the touch.
- Later the kitten becomes weak, stops crying and is uncoordinated. Sucking is weak or stops entirely.
- The queen rejects the kitten.
- The kitten's temperature is 35°C (95°F) or less.

Action

- *Slow, gentle* heating, for example, with a hot water bottle, can lead to full recovery within 24 hours.

Caution

- Take care not to warm the kitten rapidly as this can lead to shock and death.

Paralysis

Severe traumas, such as those caused by motor vehicle accidents, are common sources of spinal injury and paralysis.

Signs

- If the cat cannot use the hind limbs and there is no pulling away of the limbs when the toes are pinched, suspect a middle to lower spinal injury.
- If the cat cannot use the forelimbs and hind limbs and there is no response to pinching the toes, suspect a head or neck injury.

Action

- If the cat is lying quietly, place a flat board alongside and gently pull the cat to bring the cat onto the board, avoiding pressure on the spinal column or neck.
- Alternatively, gently pull the cat onto a blanket or towel

placed alongside. With one person at each end to hold the corners, the blanket or towel can be used as a stretcher to lift and carry the cat (see page 19).
•Take the cat to your veterinarian.

Caution

• Transport the cat with minimal movement of the spine to prevent any further damage to the spinal cord.

Penis Blocked

Causes

• A blocked penis is not uncommon among cats, and can be fatal.
• Sand-like crystals, consisting mainly of a magnesium compound called struvite, form in the urine. The male cat's urethra is long and narrow and has a bend in it, which is readily blocked.
• The condition includes inflammation of the bladder and urethra.
• A blocked penis may result from one or more of the following:
- Infection.
- Alkaline urine.
- Excessive amounts of magnesium in the diet.
- Restricted access to water.
- Excessive amounts of dry food.
- Reduced physical activity.
- Restricted access to the place where the cat normally urinates, causing retention of stale urine in the bladder for lengthy periods of time.

Signs

• Squatting frequently.
• Straining to urinate (often mistaken for constipation).
• Licking around the penis.
• Urinating in unusual places.

- Blood in urine.
- Crying in pain, especially when picked up.
- Lethargy.
- Not eating; swollen abdomen.
- Suffering from shock.
- End of penis, if protruding, may be red to bluish in colour.

Action

- Contact your veterinarian immediately. If treatment is delayed, a blocked penis can be fatal because of build-up of toxic waste products in the blood or rupture of the bladder.

Prevention

- Ensure that the cat has access to clean water at all times.
- Increase the cat's fluid intake by adding water and a small amount of salt to the diet.
- Take the cat off dry food—even though dry cat food now has a reduced amount of magnesium.
- Provide the cat with a clean litter tray or ready access to the garden.
- Encourage the cat to exercise.
- Your veterinarian can provide a prescription diet which will dissolve the struvite crystals that have formed in the bladder. After two to three months the crystals will be completely dissolved. The veterinarian will then prescribe another diet, which will prevent crystals from reforming by keeping the urine acidic and the magnesium level low. Keep your cat permanently on this prescription diet.

Poisoning

Causes

- Cats are generally very careful about what they eat.
- Cats are inquisitive, hunting animals by nature and so are quite likely to be bitten by poisonous creatures.
- Cats confined to their own homes can be exposed to

such household poisons as disinfectants, insecticidal
sprays, herbicides, pesticides, kerosene or paint.
• Cats can be poisoned inadvertently as a result of the
owner not following instructions on an insecticidal rinse
container.
• In cases of contamination of the cat's coat with a toxic
substance, the poison is taken in not so much through
the skin as by ingestion when the cat licks the coat to
clean itself.
• Some drugs, such as aspirin, can be lethal to cats,
although perfectly safe if the correct dose is administered.

Signs

• The common signs are abdominal pain, salivating,
vomit which may be blood-tinged, lethargy, diarrhea,
burns about the mouth, reddening of the skin,
staggering, twitching, depression, convulsions and coma.
Only one or a few of these signs may be evident because
they vary according to the type of poison, the quantity
ingested and the length of time that the cat has been
poisoned.

Action

• Telephone your veterinarian and describe the signs if
you are not sure of what has poisoned your cat. Some
countries have local poison information centres that can
also provide assistance.
• Initiate treatment *if you are sure* that the cat has been
poisoned and you have identified the poison involved.
• The treatment will vary according to the poison
involved. See pages 80-85 for specific treatments of
poisoning. See pages 54-57 for bites.

1. Induce vomiting

Only induce vomiting for certain poisons (see pages 80-
85), and if the cat is conscious and able to vomit. If the
cat is unconscious or semiconscious when induced to
vomit, it may inhale some of the vomit into the lungs
causing death by asphyxiation or inhalation pneumonia.

Give the cat Syrup of Ipecac (average adult dose is 2mls per kg (2.2lb) of the cat's body weight). An alternative is 10 to 20mls (2 to 4 teaspoons) of a saltwater solution, concentration 3 teaspoons of salt to half a cup of warm water.

2. Wash the cat

Only wash the cat for certain poisons (see pages 80-85). If the cat's hair and skin are contaminated with a poisonous substance, wash with warm water and soap, then rinse several times with plain water.

3. Give the cat water to drink

If the cat has taken the poison internally via the mouth, give copious amounts of water to drink. In the case of an acid, give sodium bicarbonate (baking soda) solution if readily available. Where kerosene or phenol is ingested, 2 tablespoons of olive oil by mouth are recommended.

4. Special treatment

Consult you veterinarian about medical oxygen or antidotes. See page 44 for resuscitation technique.

Convulsions

• If the cat is convulsing intermittently, wait until the convulsions stop, then take the cat to your veterinarian together with a sample of the suspected poison if available (see page 15 for handling, lifting and carrying).
• If the cat is convulsing continuously, try to save the cat from self-injury by providing protective padding, for example, a folded blanket under the head. Avoid being bitten. Contact your veterinarian immediately for advice.

Using the poisons table

To use the following table , you must be sure that your cat has been poisoned and know what poison is involved before giving treatment. If uncertain, contact a veterinarian or poison information centre immediately.

SPECIFIC TREATMENT FOR POISONS FOUND IN THE HOME AND GARDEN

Poison	Sources
Acids	Battery acids
Alcohol—Methylated spirits	An irresponsible person may offer alcohol to a cat.
Anti-freeze (Ethylene glycol)	Used in car radiators; some cats like taste, will seek out and drink.
Arsenic (vermin, poisons, insecticides, herbicides)	Ingestion of grass sprayed or rodents poisoned with arsenical preparations; licking fur covered with insecticidal or herbicidal spray.
Aspirin (Acetylsalicylic acid)	Usually administered by owner without veterinary advice to alleviate pain or discomfort—a single large dose or a series of small doses can be poisonous.
Barbiturates, Sedatives, Anti-depressants	Sleeping tablets; valium.
Benzine hexachloride (Lindane, Dieldrin, Aldrin, Chlordane, Gammexane)	Insecticidal rinse for cats in concentrated form.
Carbon monoxide	Car exhaust fumes; cat exposed to fumes if kept in garage.

Signs *(in order of onset or severity)*	Treatment
Burns on skin and mouth; vomiting may contain blood; shock.	If on skin, wash with warm water and soap, and rinse thoroughly and repeatedly with water. If ingested *do not* induce vomiting; give sodium bicarbonate (baking soda) in water and contact your veterinarian immediately.
Depression; wobbling; vomiting; collapse.	Give water; keep cat warm; contact your veterinarian.
Wobbling; vomiting; depression; convulsions; coma.	If sure that cat has ingested anti-freeze, induce vomiting (see page 79); take cat to your veterinarian who will inject ethyl alcohol to block effect of anti-freeze and administer further supportive treatment.
Salivating; thirsty; vomiting; fluid diarrhea with blood; abdominal pain; collapse; death.	Induce vomiting in early stages (see page 79); contact your veterinarian immediately who will administer antidote.
Signs vary according to period of time during which dosage administered—include poor appetite; depression; pale gums; vomiting; blood-tinged vomitus; staggering; falling over.	If recently administered, induce vomiting (see page 79); give sodium bicarbonate (baking soda) solution by mouth; contact your veterinarian.
Depression; wobbling; coma.	In early stages, induce vomiting (see page 79); contact your veterinarian.
Agitated; restless; twitching; convulsions; coma; death.	If no sign of convulsions, wash with soap and water and rinse thoroughly; contact your veterinarian.
Legs wobbly; breathing difficult; gums and mucous membrane around eyes (conjunctiva) bright pink.	Remove cat from poisonous environment to fresh air; if not breathing, give artificial respiration (see page 44); contact your veterinarian immediately who can administer oxygen directly to lungs with an endotracheal tube and give a respiratory stimulant.

SPECIFIC TREATMENT FOR POISONS FOUND IN THE HOME AND GARDEN

Poison	Sources
Chlorine	Concentrated powder or tablet used in swimming pools — chlorinated swimming pool water is not poisonous.
Kerosene	Heating fuel and cleaning fluid has a burning effect on cat's skin; cat licks affected area, thereby ingesting kerosene orally.
Lead	No longer used in paint manufacture, but some old houses still covered with lead paint; soil around lead mines polluted with lead; cat becomes poisoned by licking its coat contaminated with lead.
Metaldehyde	Snail and slug poison in powder or pellet form; cats like the taste and actively seek it out.
Oil, grease	Cat lying under a motor vehicle or accidentally falling into a container.
Organo-phosphate carbomate	Snail and slug poison in pellet form; some cats like the taste and will actively seek it out.
Paracetamol	Household pain reliever; may be administered to cat by owner.
Phenol (carbolic acid)	A potent disinfectant; poisonous to cats by ingestion or absorption through skin; after skin contact, cat may ingest by licking the contaminated hair and skin.

Signs *(in order of onset or severity)*	Treatment
Weeping red eyes; salivating; red mouth; ulcerations of mouth and tongue; vomiting; diarrhea.	Rinse eyes and mouth with water; encourage cat to drink water; contact your veterinarian.
Red, inflamed skin; vomiting; diarrhea; possible convulsions; inflamed and ulcerated tongue.	Wash the cat's skin with soap and water; give it 20–30ml (2 tablespoons) of olive oil; contact your veterinarian.
Poor appetite; weight loss; vomiting; anaemic; diarrhea. Depending on degree of lead poisoning, cat may show signs of hyperexcitability, convulsions, depression, blindness, paralysis, coma.	Lead poisoning shows up over a period of time; consult your veterinarian who will confirm lead poisoning by a blood or urine test and will treat your cat with an antidote as well as for any presenting symptoms.
Tremor; salivation; diarrhea; wobbling; convulsions.	If cat observed at time of ingestion, induce vomiting (see page 79); contact your veterinarian immediately; recovery rate very good.
Covered in grease or oil; depressed.	Wash with warm water and soap; if unable to remove oil or grease, see your veterinarian.
Tremor; salivation; diarrhea; wobbling; convulsions.	If observed at time of ingestion, induce vomiting (see page 79); contact your veterinarian immediately; recovery rate very good.
May appear hours to days after ingestion. Include lethargy; gums may range from pale (anaemic) to yellow (jaundiced) to bluish; difficult breathing; swelling of lips and face.	Induce vomiting if recently ingested (see page 79); contact your veterinarian.
Cat smells of phenol; vomiting; diarrhea; severe abdominal pain; shock; collapse.	Remove phenol from hair and skin with soap and warm water; give 20–30ml (2 tablespoons) of olive oil by mouth; contact your veterinarian.

SPECIFIC TREATMENT FOR POISONS FOUND IN THE HOME AND GARDEN

Poison	Sources
Strychnine	Rat poison, often used deliberately to poison animals with a bait.
Thallium	Rat, cockroach and ant poisons; cat can be poisoned by eating poisoned rat.
Turpentine (turps)	Paint solvent, wrongly used to remove paint from cat's hair or to dab on tick embedded in skin. Never use turps on cat's hair or skin as it can poison by absorption through skin.
Warfarin	The cat may eat the poison itself or eat a dead rat that has been poisoned with warfarin, which stops blood from clotting.

Signs *(in order of onset or severity)*	Treatment
Restless; twitching; general stiffness; convulsions with head and neck arched and limbs stretched out; convulsion can be set off by a touch or noise, become continuous, followed by death.	If cat has ingested strychnine, but shows no symptoms, induce vomiting immediately (see page 79). If showing symptoms, take to veterinarian immediately. In transit, do not touch cat or make a noise. If cat dies, strychnine can be confirmed by chemical analysis of stomach contents.
Vary according to amount ingested and period of time it is in cat's system. Redness of skin followed by a crust, peeling, and hair loss; starts on ears and lips, progresses to head, feet, limbs and body. Further symptoms are weight loss; vomiting; diarrhea; wobbling; convulsions.	Veterinarian can confirm by testing for thallium in urine. If cat has just swallowed thallium, induce vomiting (see page 79); see your veterinarian who will administer a drug to bind thallium and prevent its absorption through intestine.
Red, inflamed skin; cat vigorously licks skin affected by turps; vomiting; diarrhea; abdominal pain; restlessness; hyper-excitable; wobbly; coma.	Wash skin and hair with soap and water, rinse thoroughly; see your veterinarian.
Lethargy; pale gums and membrane around eye; weakness; laboured breathing; may be signs of haemorrhage in gum tissue; collapse; death. Signs may be slow to develop and vary according to time and amount ingested.	If recently ingested, induce vomiting (see page 79); treat for shock (see page 86); see your veterinarian who can administer an antidote; recovery rate very good.

Prevention

- Make certain that all toxic substances are kept out of reach.
- Use only clean containers for the cat's food and drinking bowls.
- In laying baits for vermin, slugs and snails or spraying the garden with herbicides and pesticides, make sure that your cat has no access to the areas concerned while the products are toxic.

Shock

Causes

- Shock is a term used to describe a state of collapse.
- Shock may range from mild to severe, and can bring about total collapse, coma and death.
- Shock usually results from some physical trauma often associated with blood loss, poison, infection or dehydration.
- Shock is often evident in accident cases.

Signs

- Weakness, lying down.
- Rapid, weak pulse.
- Pale gums and conjunctiva.
- Rapid, shallow breathing.
- Cold to the touch.

Action

- Calm the cat (see page 14).
- Keep the cat warm, to maintain normal body temperature, by wrapping the cat in a blanket and/or by using a hot water bottle or heating pad.
- Control any bleeding (see page 58).
- In cases of other than mild shock, take the cat to your veterinarian for immediate treatment.

Wounds

• Most wounds in cats are contaminated and, as such, antibiotic treatment by your veterinarian should be considered.
• Wounds are classified as abrasions, contusions, incised wounds, lacerations and puncture wounds.

ABRASIONS
Signs

• The normal abrasion is painful to the touch, haemorrhages a little and more often than not is contaminated with debris.
• The hair and surface layer of skin, and sometimes the underlying tissue, are removed.

Action

• Clean the wound by spraying or by running water from a hose onto it. Water pressure should be sufficient to wash out debris but not so strong as to drive the debris into the damaged tissue. Alternatively, clean the wound initially with 3% hydrogen peroxide.
• When the wound is clean, pat it dry with clean gauze and dust or spray it with an antibiotic.
• Leave the abrasion open to the air to dry, but if oozing freely, cover it with a gauze pad and bandage, and finally with an adhesive bandage until the oozing stops (see page 25).
• If the abrasion is left exposed to the air, use an Elizabethan collar (see page 30) so that the cat cannot lick the wound.

Caution

• If the abrasion is deep, exposing bone, tendons and so on, contact your veterinarian immediately.
• Vigorous and frequent licking of the wound will irritate it and slow down or prevent its healing.

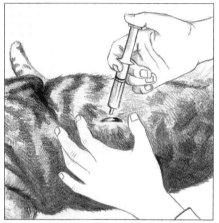

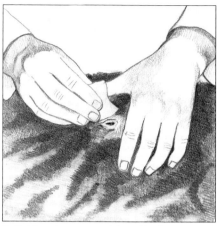

1. A wound can be cleaned by flushing with 3% hydrogen peroxide from a syringe.

2. Pat the clean wound dry with clean gauze.

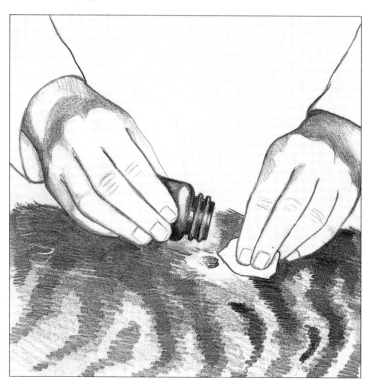

3. Dust the wound with an antibiotic powder or spray.

• These wounds are characterised by bruising and
swelling of the skin and underlying tissue. They are not
necessarily associated with a break in the skin.
• Caused by a kick, fall or collision.

• If there is a break in the skin, see your veterinarian who
will administer antibiotics.

• If there is no break in the skin and you are aware of the
contusion immediately after it occurs, apply a cold
compress. A swelling that has been present for some time
and feels firm to hard is best dealt with by applying a hot
foment (compress).

Cold compress Hose the swollen area with a fair
amount of water pressure or apply an icepack for 30
minutes. The cold constricts the blood vessels and the
pressure has a massaging effect.

Hot foment (compress) Pour hot water into a bucket
containing 2 tablespoons of salt. The temperature of the
water should be so hot that you can *just* put your hand
into the water and keep it there. Soak a large wad of
cottonwool (absorbent cotton) in the hot solution, then
hold it on the contused area until it cools off. Repeat for
five minutes twice daily. The heat dilates the blood
vessels helping to soften and disperse the swelling.

• The characteristics of these wounds are clean-cut, fairly
well opposed edges and minimum tissue damage.
• Caused by broken glass or similar sharp objects.

• If bleeding, apply pressure directly to the wound with a
clean gauze pad or similar until the bleeding stops.
• Clean the wound only if necessary.
• Gently but firmly pinch the opposing edges of the
wound together (see page 91).
• Apply thin strips of adhesive bandage in a crisscross

formation about 1cm (0.5in) apart directly across the wound.
• Place a gauze pad over the wound. Secure with a gauze bandage held in place by an adhesive bandage. This will help to immobilise the edges of the wound (see page 25).
• Confine the cat.
• Leave the bandage in place for 48 hours, then check the wound.
• If the wound is clean, dry and showing no sign of inflammation, rebandage and change every 48 hours.

Caution

• If the wound is extensive (long and/or deep), contact your veterinarian to have it stitched.
• Such a wound should be stitched within eight hours.

LACERATIONS
Signs

• The wound edges are often irregular, jagged and gaping. Sometimes whole sections of the skin and underlying tissue are torn away.
• Lacerations are usually not painful and haemorrhage is variable.
• Caused by barbed wire, sharp edge of a tin, and so on.

Action

• Thoroughly clean the wound by hosing it or by applying 3% hydrogen peroxide.
• Remove any hair, dead tissue or foreign bodies from the wound.
• Apply antibiotic powder.
• Cover the wound with a gauze pad then a gauze bandage, both held firmly in place by an adhesive bandage (see page 25).
• See your veterinarian as the laceration may need to be stitched.
• If unable to be stitched, leave the bandage in place for two days.
• When the bandage is removed, hose the wound to clean away any discharge, debris or dead tissue and dress the wound as before.

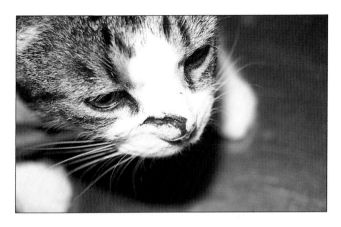

1. An incised wound on the cat's nose.

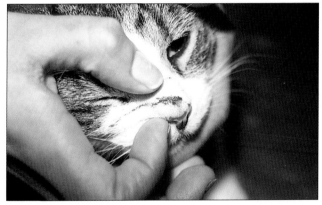

2. The opposing edges of the wound are gently but firmly pinched together.

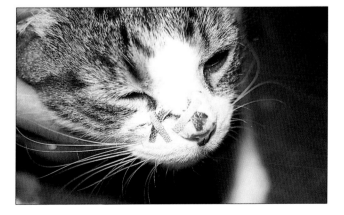

3. Crisscross strips of adhesive tape hold the wound edges together.

• Continue the bandaging until fleshy tissue has filled in the cavity to skin level. Then leave the bandage off, allowing the air and sunshine to dry the surface of the wound.
• If the cat licks the wound excessively, apply an Elizabethan collar (see page 30).
• Restrict exercise until the skin has completely covered the wound.

PUNCTURE WOUNDS

• Puncture wounds are generally painful and may or may not be accompanied by haemorrhage.
• Can be caused by eye tooth penetration in a fight or penetration of the skin by a splinter, piece of wire or nail.

Action

• Carefully clip the hair away from the hole.
• Carefully check the wound to see that no foreign body remains embedded.
• Clean the area with 3% hydrogen peroxide and dab the wound with tincture of iodine.
• Do not allow a seal to form. Keep the wound open as long as possible while drainage is taking place.
• If the puncture appears to penetrate through the skin into the underlying tissue, take the cat to your veterinarian who will administer antibiotics and if necessary drain the wound.

INDEX

ACKNOWLEDGMENTS

I would like to thank my wife Jan and children Melanie, Samantha, Damien and Edwina for being so patiently supportive during the time of writing.

My sincere thanks to my father Eric for his diligent assistance in planning, researching and proofreading, and also to my sister Judy Shields for undertaking the daunting task of deciphering my notes and transferring them to print.

I would also like to thank my partner Dr David Lonergan and the staff of Gordon Veterinary Hospital — Dr Andrew Morgan, Dr Sue McMillan and the nurses, Jenifer Reber, Kim Tupper and Diane Spalding — for their kindly advice and generous spirit of co-operation.

TIM HAWCROFT